Prelude

This story starts a long time ago, June 13th, 1948, only 3 years after the end of World War 2. That was the day I was born. I can't remember where exactly, I just remember I was there when it happened. I do know that I grew up in a small "village", Tower Gardens" in East Lansing, Mi., a place and time where everybody knew everybody else, where nobody locked their doors, and kids actually played Outdoors. Imagine, no computers, no electronic games, no cell phones and texting every where. Kids rode bikes, just for the fun of it, with a playing card stuck in the spokes making a rapid clack clack clack sound. That was supposed to sound like a motorcycle engine. I grew up with all these things, and a lot more, many things never even heard of by todays generations.

   I spent most of my youth in Tower Gardens, and learned a lot of things there. I learned how to street fight the neighborhood bully, I learned how to ride my first bike, which Dad got from a friend, I learned you do Not open a pressure cooker full of greens until it has fully cooled and has no pressure left inside, what a mess. I learned how to kiss, and liked it, a lot, and I learned how to smoke, at the ripe old age of 15. It started when my Uncle Guy came over to the house, and I spotted a pack of Pall Malls, unfiltered, on the car seat. I didn't think he would miss them, so I took them. I thought I was really "cool" then. I showed my neighbors, who happend to be my 3rd cousins. They were 2 girls, and another girl friend of theirs, who 's name I have forgotten since then. I do remember she liked to kiss as much as I did, and we spent a lot of time with our lips locked together. I should have stuck with the kissing, and left the cigarettes alone, but instead, we looked for some matches. I thought my head was going to come off, I coughed so hard after that first drag, but went back for more, all of us laughing, coughing, and maybe turning a little green. That pack of smokes lasted us a couple weeks.

   It wasn't until many years later that I started smoking heavy. My Mom smoked, and I would swipe a single cigarette out of a pack now and then. This went on for a couple years, until I got my first job, and managed to buy my own. I used to hide them under the back porch while at home. It wasn't until I went in the Army that I "came out" as a smoker. That was 1968, 44 years ago. I smoked for 40 years, smoking more and more all the time. It was probably 20 years after I started that I started feeling the effects, tiredness, out of breath easily, a cough that just stayed with me. Eventually, I went to see a doctor. He told me that if I didn't stop smoking, in a couple more years I would be on oxygen. I just brushed that aside. Turns out he was right. I was up to almost 3 packs a day, smoking even when I coughed so hard I could hardly take a drag. Between 10-12 years ago I was told I had COPD, and Emphyzema, and was put on Oxygen, only as needed at first, then full time as I got worse. Almost 4 years ago my wife, Connie, and I quit smoking, together. About 2 years ago, or so, I was referred to a Lung Dr. in Ann Arbor, Dr Chan. I was diagnosed with End Stage Emphyzema, and was told I had only 3 years left to live. I asked him about a Lung Reduction, and was told that was not an option, but maybe a whole Lung Transplant. I was put through extensive testing, and found I was eligible for a double lung transplant. I was put on a waiting list, where I remained for 1 year, 4 months. Just when I thought I would never get "the call", it happened. What follows is a journal, and some pictures, put together from notes and pictures that my wife, Connie, and sister Debbie, put together. There is so much more I probably could have included, but I didn't want to get too boring.

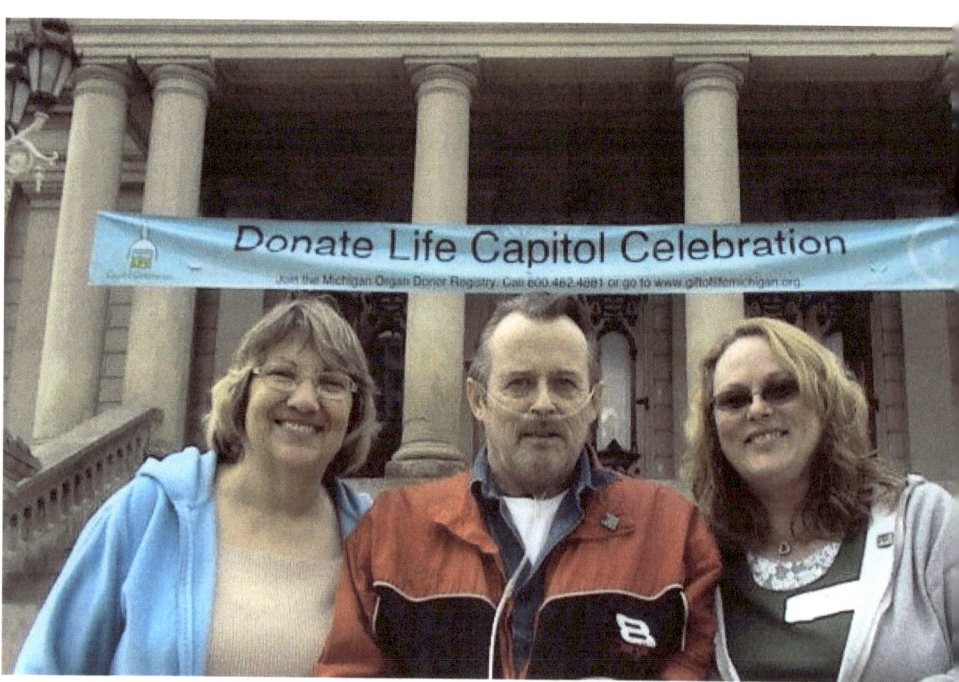

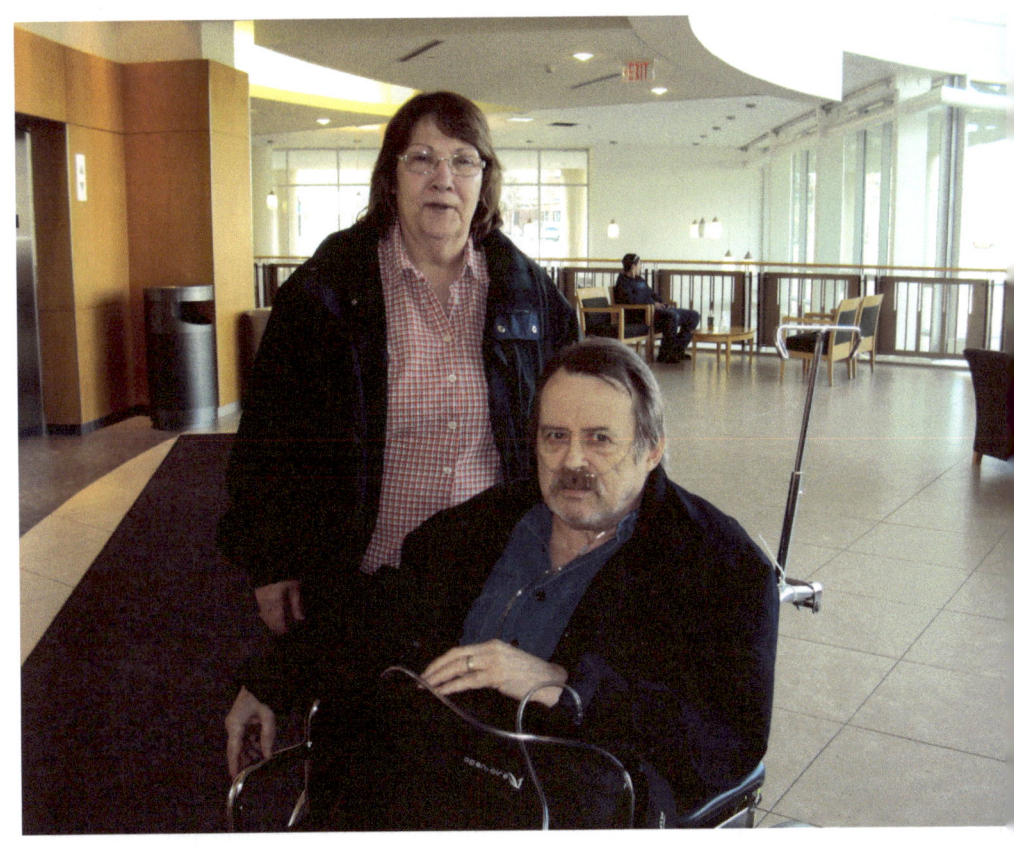

Double Lung Transplant

September 2010 seen Dr. Chang

November 23, 2010 was put on the donor list

April 2, 2012 received call for double lung transplant

It was Monday, April 2, 2012 approx. 7:30 a.m., when U of M called to tell me they had a set of lungs for me. I couldn't believe it; I had to have them repeat it. Connie had already left for work so I called her right away and of course she was instantly on her way home. While I was waiting for her, I began to gather the things we had planned on taking, and made a few more calls to let people know that today might be the start of a new life. My sister, Debbie, went with Connie and me to U of M in Ann Arbor. I think Connie must have driven 80 mph all the way there. Debbie kept telling her to breathe and chill because we wanted to get there in one piece. After being well on our way, I realized I left my wallet at home (so I had no i.e.), we called the hospital and asked if that was going to be a problem. They told us not to worry about it. All the way there Deb was making a few more phone calls to let people know and to give them a chance to talk to me. I was facing a very big surgery. Being able to talk to family and receiving good luck wishes, and expressing the love for each other was important not only to me but for them also. Once we arrived at the hospital, (about 8:15 a.m.) We pulled up to the valet parking and were greeted immediately. When we walked inside and approached the desk, the attendant on duty greeted me by my name. Suddenly I'm famous, Ha Ha. I didn't even have to tell her who I was. She directed us to the correct floor and told us they would be waiting for me, and they were. From there they took me to my room where I would be prepped for surgery (everything had to be done as if the lungs were going to be placed in my body. What a lot to go through, knowing there was a chance that something could send me back home without getting a new set of lungs.

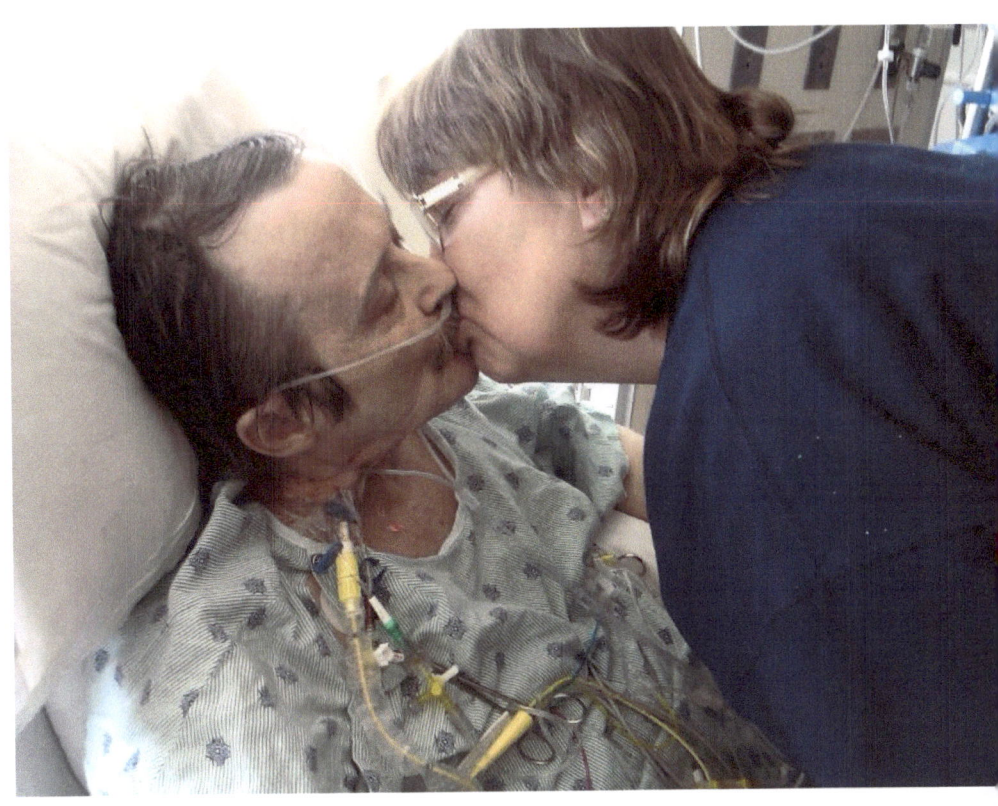

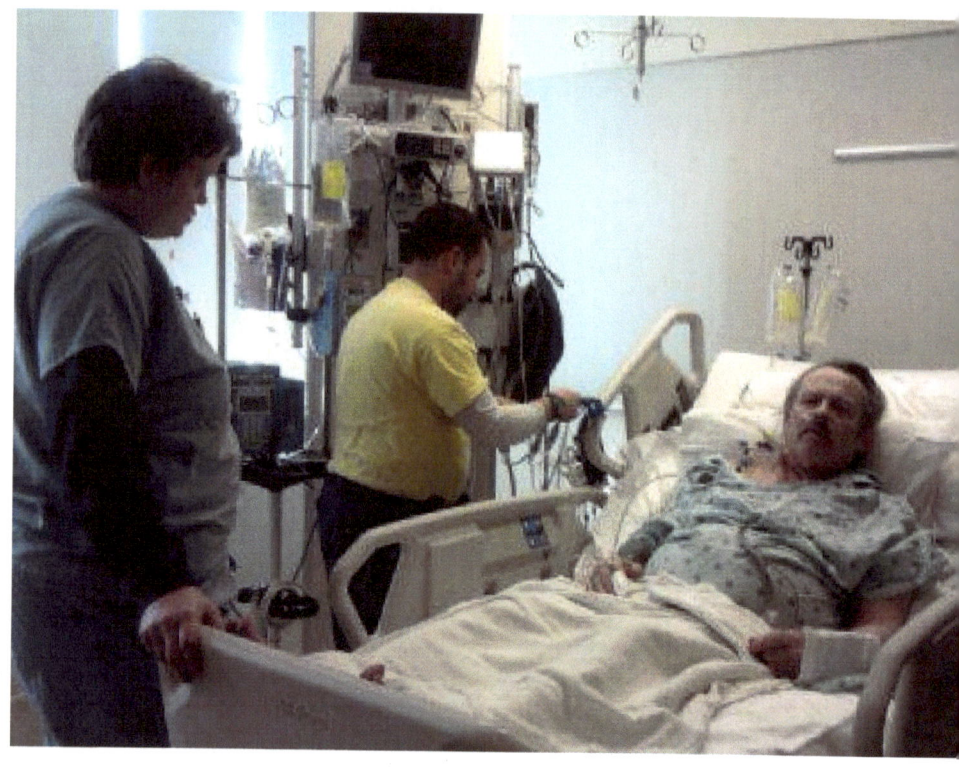

So the next several hours were spent getting into the hospital attire and getting hooked up to the monitors and I.V. Angie and Charles were the two main nurses who did everything. They helped keep the humor up by putting up with my humor. They explained everything that was going to happen and when it was going to happen. As the day progressed, nurses, doctors, anesthesiologists and anyone else who felt they needed to—came in and gave me information of how the day was going to progress. During this time there were a few more phone calls to family who weren't able to talk to me earlier. We had to be realistic, this could be what they call a "dry run" and I would just go home, or, this could be real and the surgery was going to happen. I believe it was approximately 4:00 p.m. when they were ready to take me back to surgery. It was time to give the kisses and hugs and say "I Love You". One of the last things I said was "pray for the doctors, they are the ones that have to do all the work. They are facing a 12 hour surgery; I just have to lay there". As I was being transported to surgery, my thoughts were on Connie, and the rest of my family, beginning a long night in the waiting room. Once in the operating room, my wait began. The new lungs were being tested, and prepared. I was left lying on a rather uncomfortable operating table. Doctors, nurses, techs, were just some of the people there, waiting for word that the surgery would be a go. Every time the phone would ring, or whenever someone walked in, I wondered if it was about my new lungs. It seemed like I laid there forever. I had a lot of time to think about the surgery, the possible pain later, and the good effects of the surgery. The next thing I remember is waking up in ICU four days later with someone telling me to cough so they could remove the tube from my throat. The rest of this is shared by notes that Connie and Debbie wrote down. Just as I was on the way to the surgical room Deb read a text from Kris saying good luck and that he loves me.

From Debbie's and Connie's notes: The waiting now began for Connie and I in the waiting room, as well as everyone back home who was waiting for any piece of information we could share as soon as we heard anything. It seems like we spent a lot of time watching each other, staring off into space. It was time to be strong for each other. It was really happening!!. Phone calls and texts went out to everyone barely without a breath in between. Excitement filled the air, tears of joy ran down our faces, but the fear also set in, because this was a serious surgery. Now we spent a lot of time praying that Jerry was strong enough to withstand the surgery and his body wouldn't reject the new lungs. About 8:00p.m. Larry, Barb, and Rob joined us in the waiting area. Together we watched every door open and every person walk through, waiting for the one to come that would give the news of an update. Karen, Dawn, Sue, Rachael, Kathy, Daniel and Connie's mom, Ron and Sally, Brent and Deb, and many more were constantly inquiring on how Jerry was and if there were any updates.

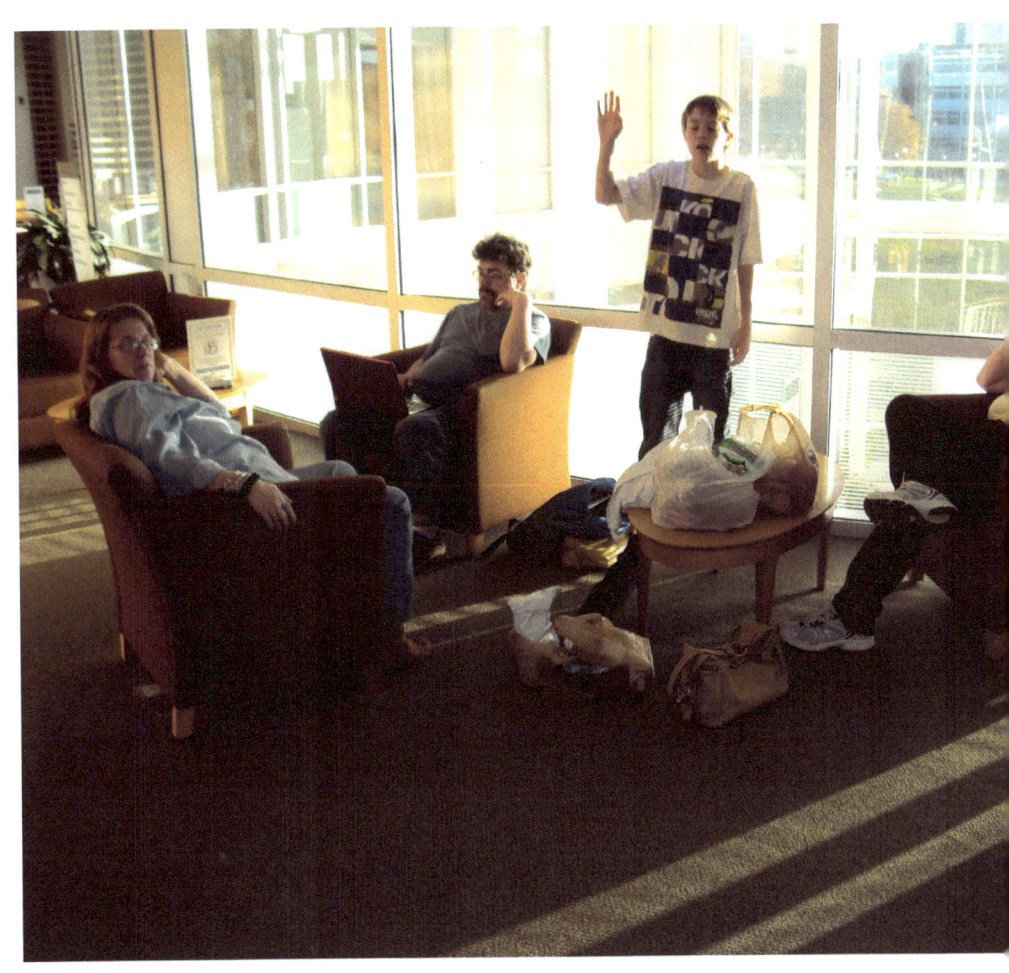

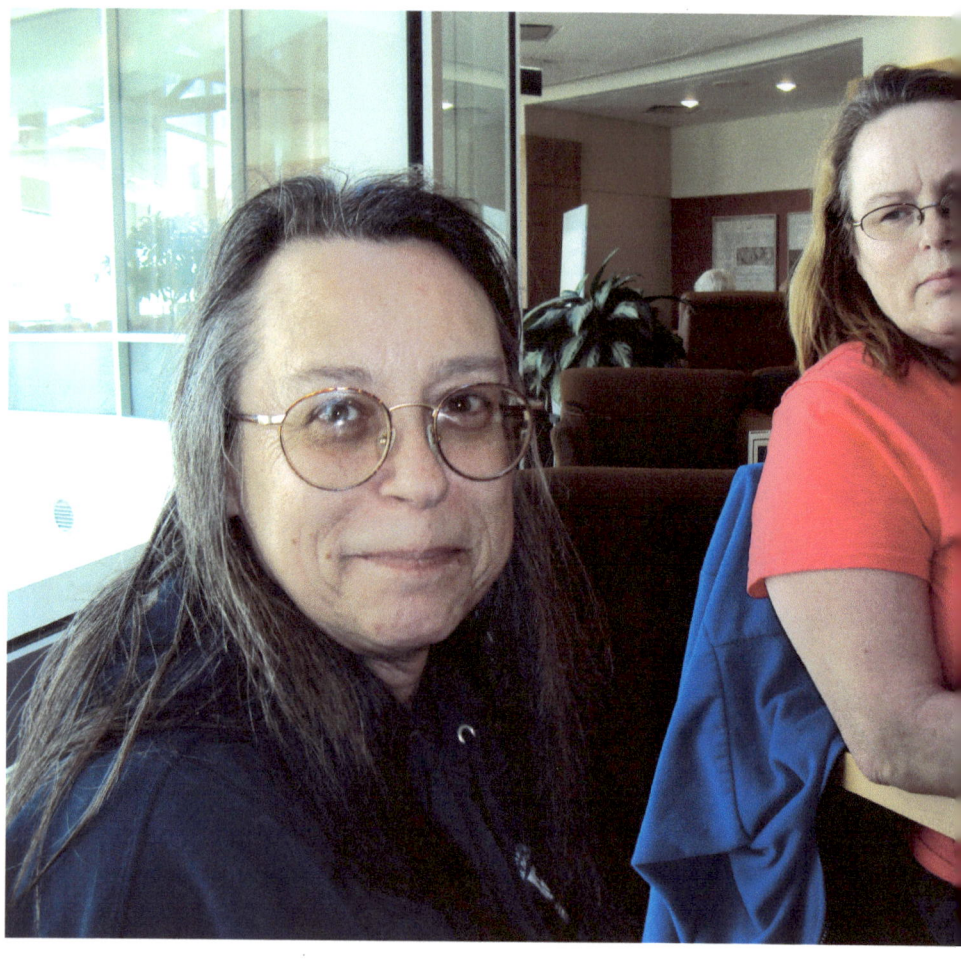

Finally about 11:00 p.m. the news came that the first lung was in and everything was going well and they were starting the second one. Larry, Barb and Rob had to work the next day so they left after getting the update. Now it was Just Connie and I again. It just so happened that I didn't have to work for a few days so I was able to stay there with Connie. So we spent the next few hours trying to get comfortable and settle in for a long night. We moved recliners around and changed spots a few times before we finally shut our eyes (we kept one eye open—waiting for the next update ...ha-ha). I think I kept my eyes open trying to make sure Connie got some sleep. About 1 a.m. or so, another nurse came out to tell us Jerry's heart was "sick". We found out later that the heart had stopped, and Jerry was put on echmo (a heart/lung bypass machine).

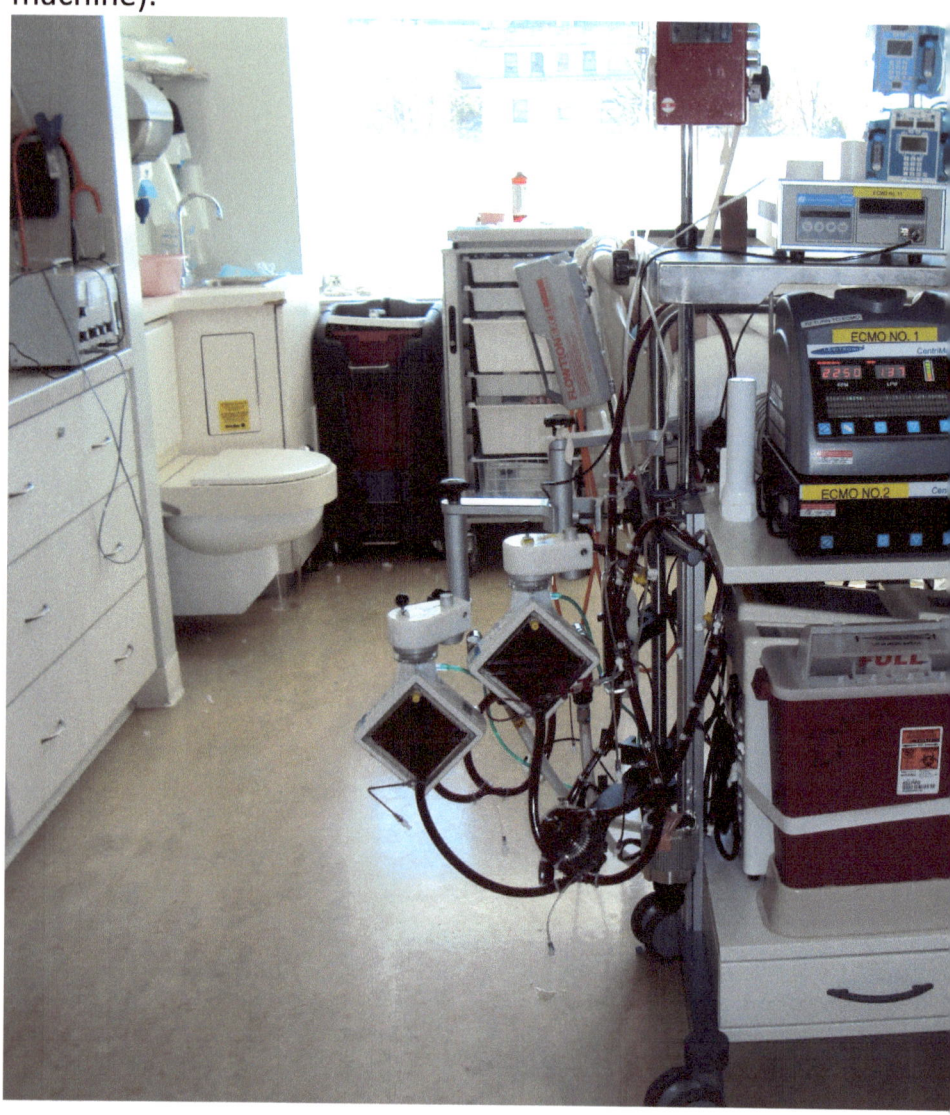

At about 3:45 a.m. the nurse came out and told us the second lung was in and you were stable. It was what she wasn't telling us that had us worried. All she would say is that you went through a lot and that the doctor would be out in a couple hours to talk to us. Well now we couldn't go back to sleep or even pretend to rest. After sending out texts and calling family we decided to hunt down the coffee and start on a puzzle. It was hard to put pieces together when the tears kept coming. There were tears of joy, of fear, of anxiety of not knowing what the doctor was going to say. Finally about 6:00 a.m. the doctor came out and took us in a private room to talk. He said this was the most difficult surgery he had ever done and he was worried, but that you were in the very best place you could be in with the very best state of the art equipment that there is, and a very good medical team watching over you. He said that your heart had stopped after getting the first lung and they had to put you on a by-pass machine. They eventually stabilized you and started the second lung and before they were able to close they had to put you back on the by-pass machine due to your heart being a bit sluggish. They never had to use the paddles to shock your heart. She said it was touch and go for a short time, but they believed considering the complications that everything went well. Your heart had stopped because of the lung going into a "sick" stage, he said that is expectable with an organ after being handled and placed into another person's body. Because your heart had went through so much, they felt it couldn't go through trying to adapt to the new lungs on its own, so they put you on what was called an "echmo by pass machine". You could be on that for a longer period of time and be on it in your room. This would give your body time to adjust and time for you to recover to where you could eventually be taken off of it. After the doctor explained everything to us he left us to comprehend it all and we cried and talked about it with each other. We helped each other understand what was just said, as we had been doing for each other all night. When one was weak, the other one was strong. We refused to believe that you weren't going to make it through this. But we had to see it for what it was. You had complications through the surgery with your heart stopping due to the lungs being traumatized during the transplant. You had to have a transfusion and you were in critical care. Your body was weak which was understandable given it had just gone through a double lung transplant and the doctor saying it was the most difficult one he had ever done.

Okay, so now, Connie and I are back on the phones, when we could keep service going. That was a challenge the entire time up there. We practically had to put our ear up to the window just to keep the signal intact. There were times that we were just talking and talking just to find out we had lost contact a few statements ago. But we were able to keep our humor, mixed in with a lot of anxiety, fear, hope, and trust in our "Father" himself that you were going to come through all this okay.

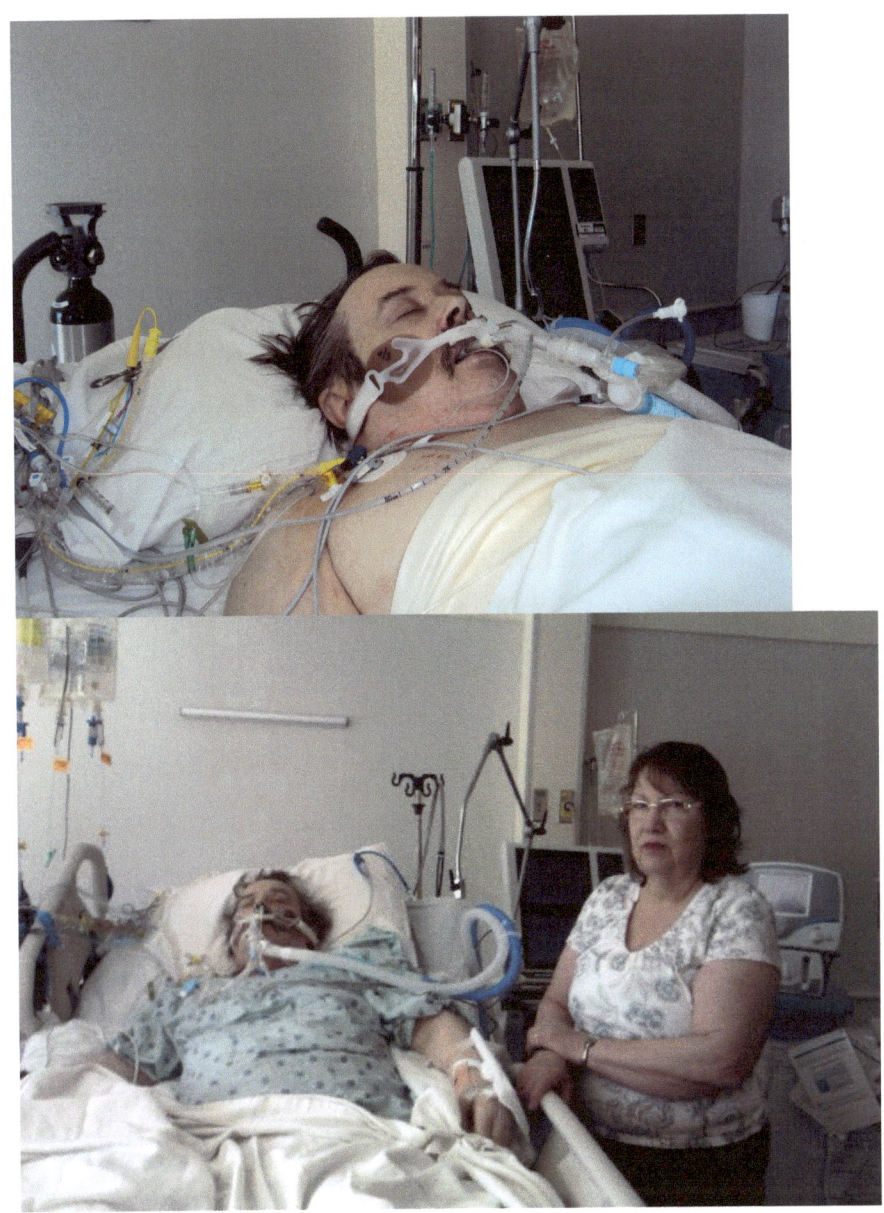

Tuesday, April3, 2012 was a long day of being with you every moment they would let us, which was any time they were not doing something in there. It was your most critical time. I couldn't have pulled Connie away even if I had wanted to. She needed to be there as much as she was allowed. You were so swollen; I said you looked like the Pillsbury doughboy. You had so many tubes and machines, lots of medicines going into you. It hardly seemed real to stand there and see you like that. Everything was working for you, keeping you alive. All the machines, leads, wires, and tubes, a lot to look at and it just made you trust with amazement that the team of doctors and nurses knew exactly what each one was and the importance of each one. Doctors said that they didn't want your heart to take on any stress while your body adapted to the lungs. So it wasn't that your heart couldn't handle it, but that it was a safety measure to ensure that your heart stayed strong for the hard fight you would have later when you would begin to wake up. That made sense, but it didn't make it any easier seeing you like that. Later, a few others came to visit. Dawn stayed the night there with Connie this time so I could go home and clean up and take care of a few things. It meant a lot that she stepped in so Connie wouldn't be there by herself. With you still being considered critical, I didn't want Connie to be by herself. Dawn and Connie got inventive with the chairs and cushions in the waiting area when it was time to get some sleep. They asked for some blankets and took several cushions from the chairs and made a bed on the floor. It made for a better nights sleeping.

On Wednesday, April 4th the doctors decided to lower the level of support to see how you would do. After three hours they felt they could take you off the by-pass. That was great news, but that meant you would be doing the work now and they would be watching you even closer. That's something we felt we never had to worry about. The nurses and doctors were constantly watching over you. You were still kept in a medical induced coma as long as you had the breathing tube in. They didn't want to take the risk of you waking up enough to realize that was still in and have you get all worked up. Now that you were off the echmo bypass their next goal was to get that breathing tube out. Before they could do that, one of your medications needed to be lowered, so that process began. Every step they took or wanted to take always depended on your progress and whether they could adjust levels of medications. They also had waiting times to see how you would handle the adjustments before they made another. Every morning, the team of doctors would make their rounds and discuss the patient's condition outside their room. Connie and I would always step out and listen when they came to you. Connie always had a question or a comment; I think the team respected her for that. Connie showed them she was knowledgeable about a lot and what she wasn't; she was going to understand by asking and being a part of your care. Sometimes the team would debate with each other on whether to change the course of treatment or to take you off a certain medication, but their goal was the same. To make sure you were tolerating anything that was done, before taking you to the next step. They had agenda's each day, but sometimes those plans got delayed because you didn't respond well enough or there were too many up's and down's. Thursday, April 5th, their goal was to get you off the breathing tube by the next day. You had to get off one medication first, in the meantime, they were going to place a feeding tube in to get you ready for some food. They would always prep their steps so they would be ready to take you to the next level. Timing and making sure you were comfortable was so important. They were also going to give you an epidural later that evening so you would not feel the discomfort when they took the tube out. So like I said, up's and down's got in the way sometimes and this was one of those times. Your platelets kept dropping down way low. So because you need the platelets to be up high in order for clotting to happen, they weren't going to proceed with any plans of removing your respirator. They wanted to keep you still and not bring you alert too much because they didn't want anything to cause you to bleed. So no more plans of removing the breathing tube or putting in the epidural. If you were responsive in any way it was more for their benefit to gather medical information and then they would give you medicine to let you go back to sleep. Every once in a while we were able to get you to squeeze our hand or you would make facial movements. You were in a "light" awareness stage, but not enough to be able to remember anything later, let alone remember who was there and who wasn't.

It's been four days now, every day Connie would be there watching you, studying you, looking for any sign of progress. I made sure she took breaks and that she kept her mind organized for what she had to do for herself. She would take time to figure the bills, make sure she had her medications, personal time for talking to family, eating, etc. Kathy was taking care of the animals and would collect the mail. She was the "go to" person for anything Connie needed from the house. More family started visiting so that helped me feel comfortable to not be there as much. Day five was pretty much like the rest of them, watching your vitals, watching your platelets (if they didn't stay above a certain number, all plans would stay on hold). They had to watch your heart rate closely as well. Many times it would go up high enough to put you into a fib. The one night I went home, you had one of those episodes, another one of those times of "ups and downs". Connie stayed in there with you all night. You responded to her voice in the way of facial expressions or sometimes you would squeeze her hand a bit. Every day seemed so long, watching, and waiting for you to wake up. We were worried, and Connie would ask the nurses, every day, how you were doing. We were so relieved when you finally started waking up. The doctors told you to breathe, and cough, so they could take the breathing tube out of your throat. You were in and out the first day, but you were slowly becoming more alert. It was so good to see you on your way back to us.

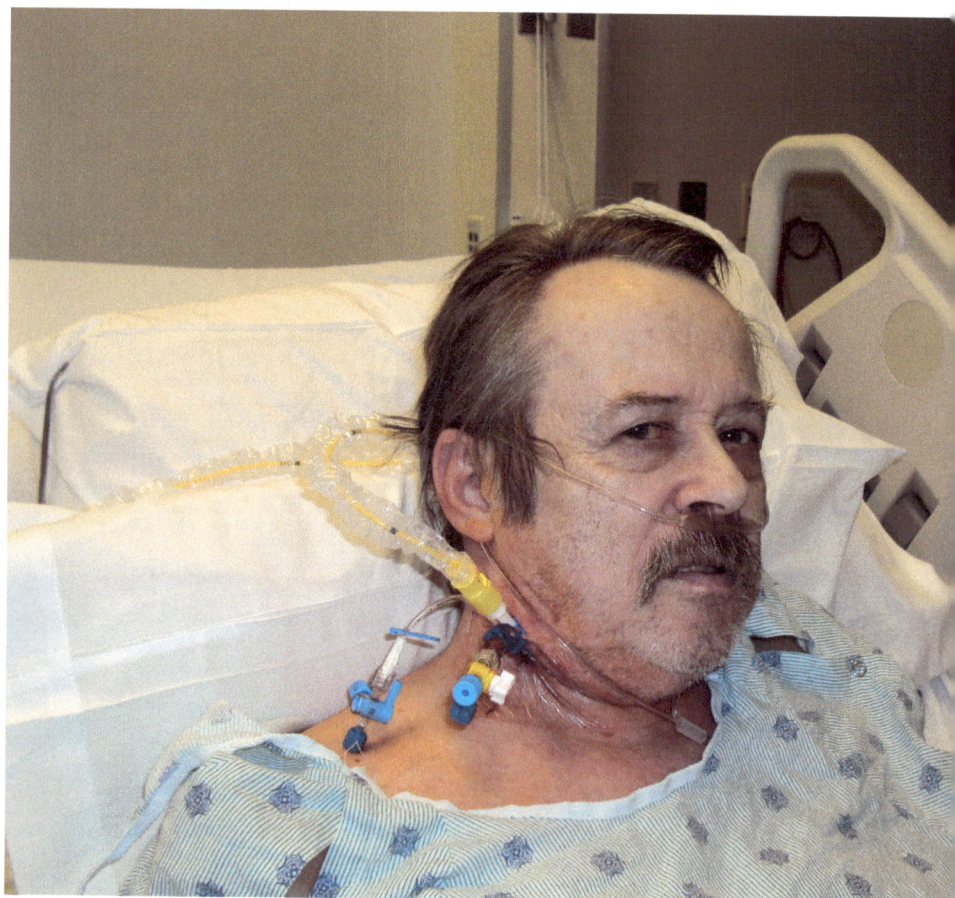

On Monday, April 9th the doctors decided they needed to move the pic line from your neck to your arm, this would allow them to still give you the medication you need in order to be taken off the ventilator and would also allow them to let you be a bit more alert. They also felt that maybe having the pic line in your neck was affecting your heart rate causing an irritability, making your rate increase. After a few hours of watching you and giving you doses of medication to help bring your rate down you finally came down where you should be. Tuesday , April 10th they moved your line to your arm, and took out one of the drain tubes. They wanted to take out the cathedar but decided it was too much too soon. So that would be the goal for the next day. Your platelets increased to 30 which was very good considering how low they have been staying. Having your platelets up is the key to what helped them make decisions for the next steps.

Me....I won't kid you, it was painful, having the chest tubes taken out, but it was over in about 5 seconds, but seemed longer. Then there is the catheter tube. Not the most pleasant thing in the world. Mine plugged up three times, I think. Very painful when pressure builds up, and you can't pee. I had to have nurse back flush it to unplug it.

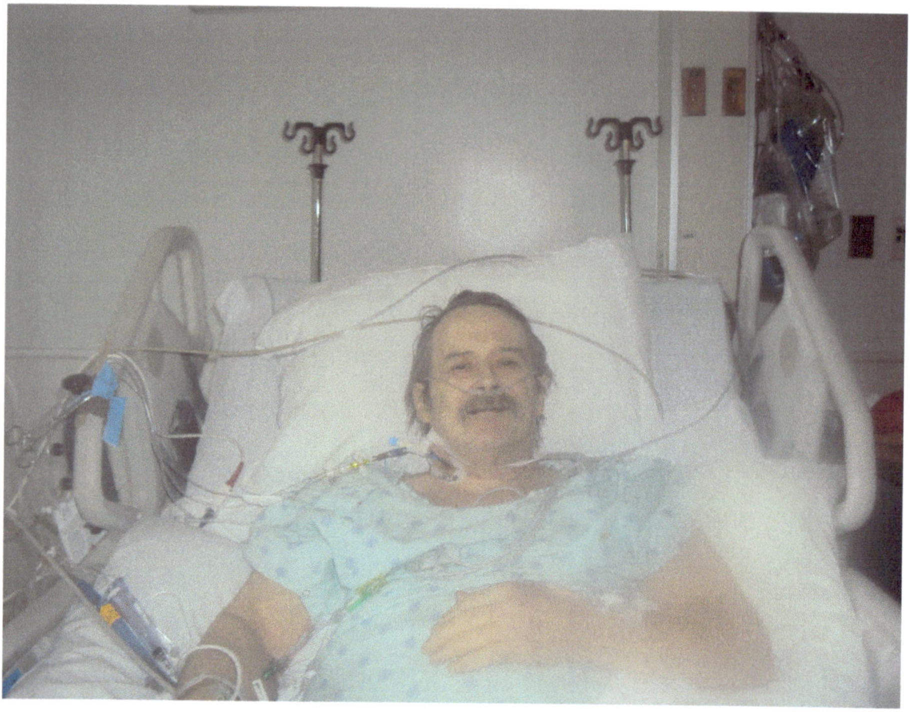

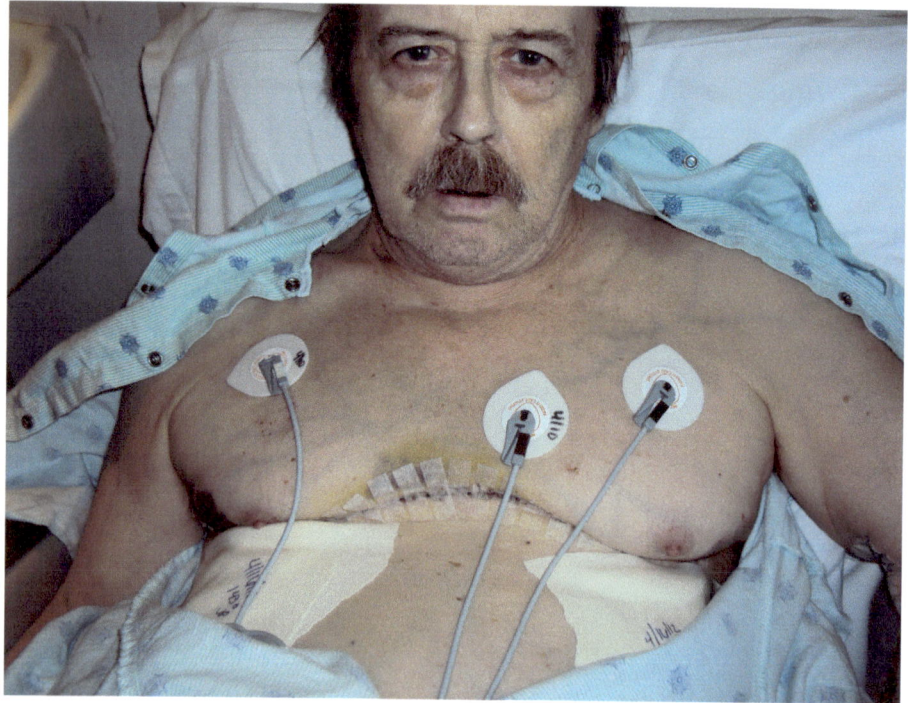

You got to sit up in the bed today and Physical therapists were going to try to get you in the chair, but during the process your heart rate went up very high again. They got you back in bed and gave you magnesium and amino to bring you back down. The doctors were very good about assuring us that even though this was serious, it was also common to see this in patients that have undergone lung transplant. So while they were amazed at the progress you were making they were also watching and waiting for the common complications to happen. They always stayed a step ahead and were ready for what your body brought to the day/to the moment. Wednesday, April 11th, they took out the two chest tubes and the catheter. That evening the night nurse (Sheila) turned your air down to one. She was very attentive and made Connie feel very comfortable. By 8:30 p.m. Your air was turned all the way off and you are doing fine. Thursday, April 12th, day nurse (Jason) started your day at 6:15 a.m., getting you up in a chair until after lunch. You were up walking at 2:30 in the hall, just a short walk. John from the support group was in to see you today, was glad to see you doing so well. Later in the day they moved you to a new room, 4448, 4th floor in the older part of the hospital. Friday , April 13th , your day nurses were Susan and Elizabeth. They got you up in a chair.

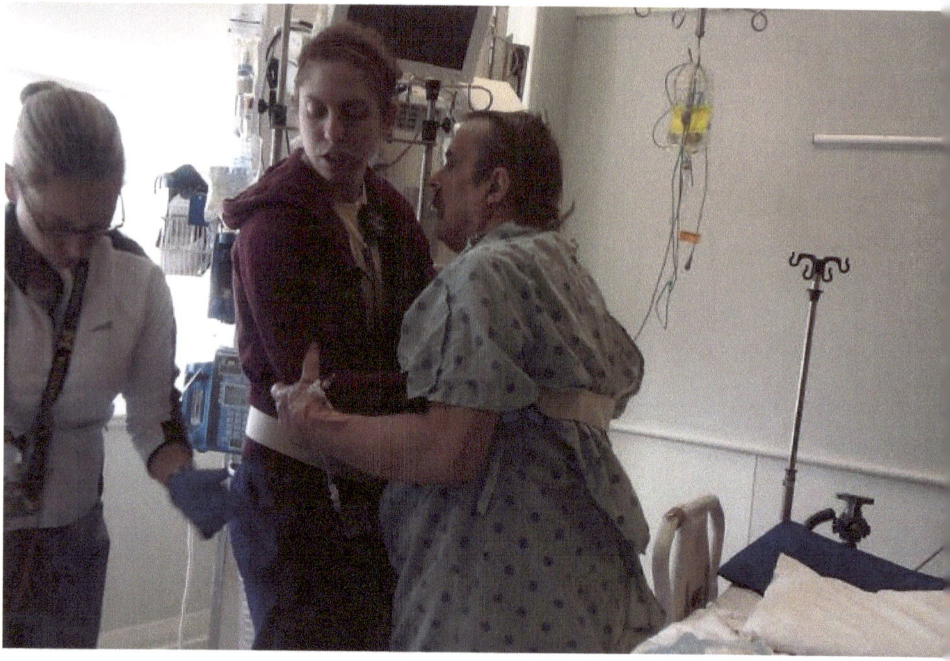

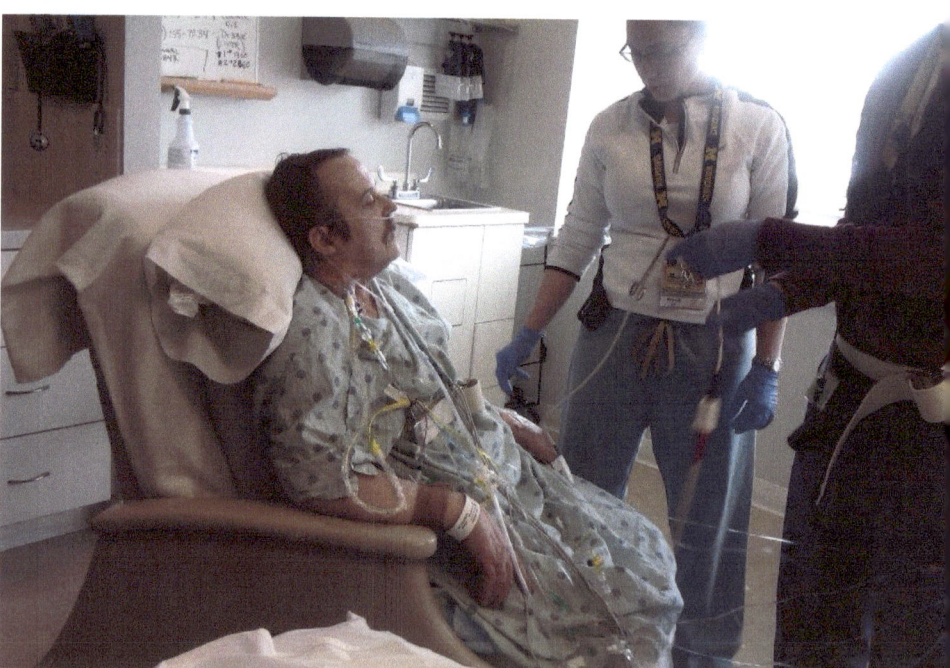

You are using the air at night while you sleep, but during the day they have you off of it. More walking and getting up out of the chair and off the bed with little assistance. You are doing very well. PT came in today about noon and walked with you. You walked about 50 feet and sat down for a few minutes. Then you walked some more, total of about 75 feet and then you were so tired that they took you back to your room in a chair. PT told you to walk at least 4 times a day up and down the hallway. Also gave you exercises to do two to three times a day, as well as your spirometer every hour. On your next walk you went about 100 feet. Third walk was 120 feet. Connie went back to her room before you did your fourth walk. She needed to get some rest and cook some chicken. She also made goulash ahead of time so she could get a quick snack.

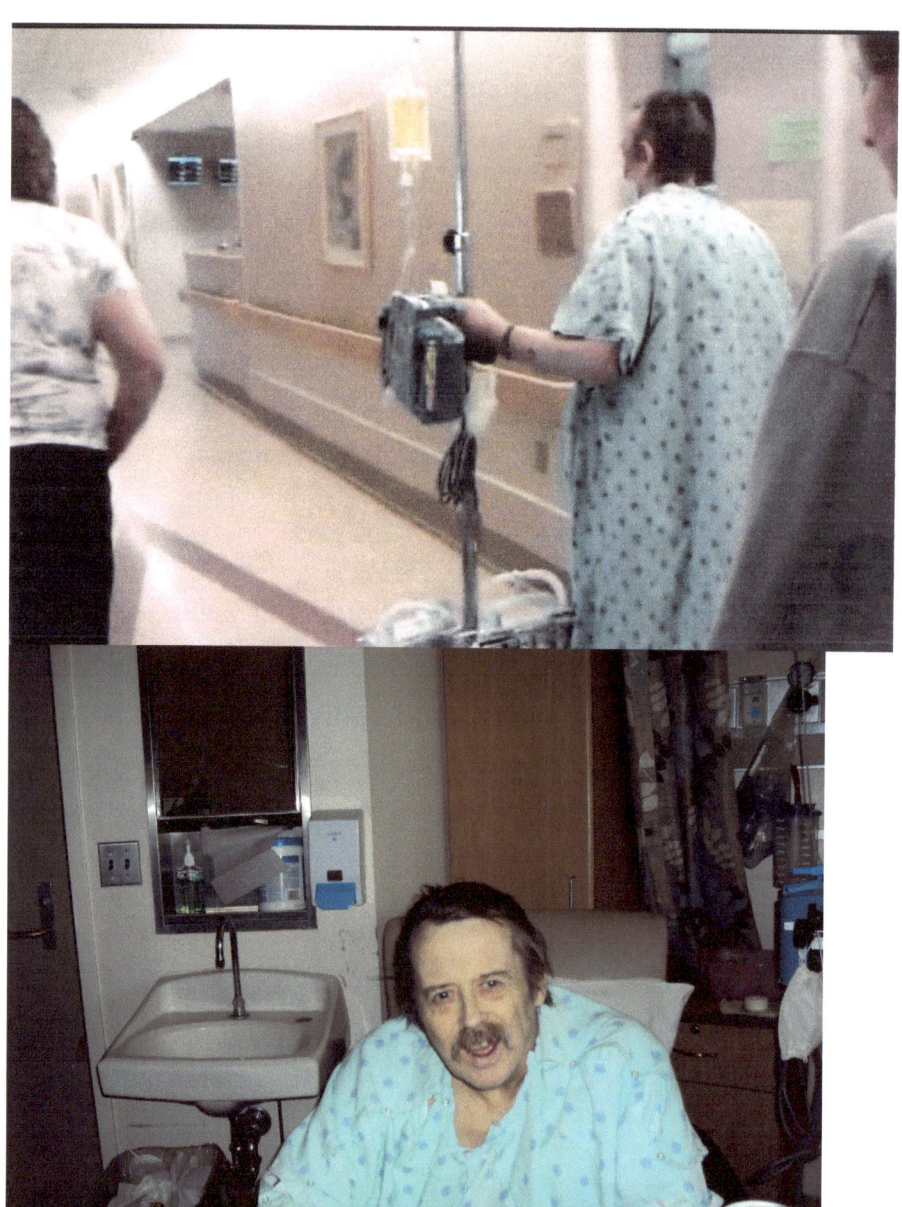

Saturday, April 14th, you were already up in the chair when Connie got there that morning. You said you didn't sleep very well. You are faithfully doing the spirometer before and after your walks, and with each walk you progress about 5 feet further. Today you had a lot of visitors. Kathy, Bud, Kay, Daniel, David, Chris, Larry, Barb, Karen, Rachael, Paige, Dan and his son was all there to see you at the same time. Everyone crowded in your room and visited with you for a while, but when they left, the nurse made it clear that from now on only three or four visitors at a time. The room was way too small for that many all at once and your immune system could easily be compromised. Later that day you and Connie watched a video about checking your sugar and got a meter kit. They trained you on how to give yourself an insulin shot and later you gave yourself your first shot in your belly.

Sunday, April 15th, you said you didn't sleep well again. You went for an X-ray today, they said the spirometer must be doing good because you started coughing phlegm up. Your first walk today went good. After your second walk they said your oxygen stayed up at 92, very good. Doctor Reddy was in and said that you were doing very good and was happy with your progress. He said that your breathing problems are because of the need for oxygen for so long that your mind thinks that you still need it. You just have to continue to train your mind that you can do this breathing on your own and remember to take deep breaths in through your nose and out your mouth. You got your last walk in for the day at 7:30 p.m. All in all, you had a good day. On Monday, April 16th, you talked to Shelly and Sharon from rehabilitation. The PT doctor came in and started you on some exercises for your hips. You were not as willing to work for Connie as you were for PT, but that's okay. They gave you a daily routine to follow, to work arms and legs sitting 2 x daily, standing working legs 2 x daily, walk at least 4 x daily and to use the spirometer every hour plus the vibro breather. The doctor said you would be two more days before he would remove any tubes. Today you worked very hard on all your exercises and ended your day falling asleep in the recliner.

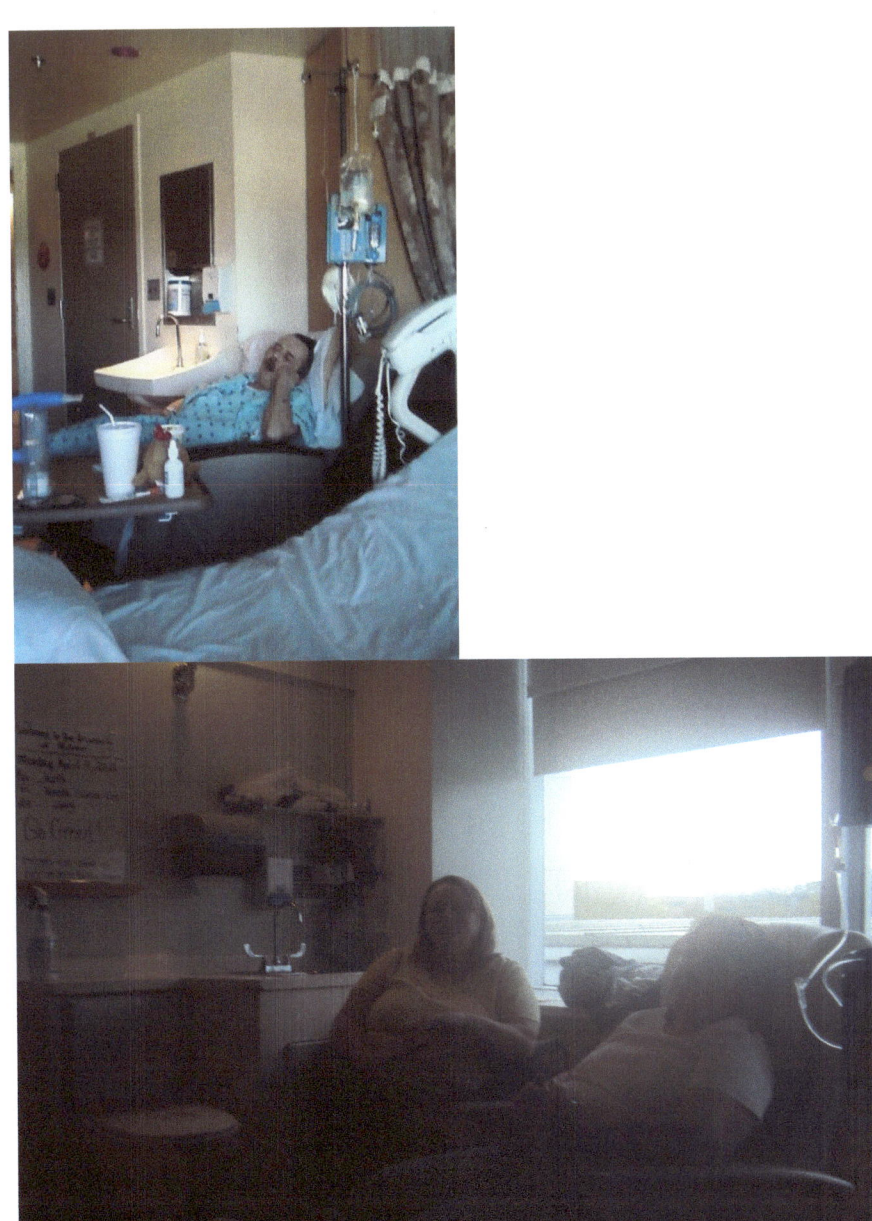

Tuesday, April 17th you went for a chest x-ray. You did some stairs with pt today, and some side steps. They told you to cough periodically through the day and to continue using the spirometer and the vibro breather. You are also continuing to learn about all your medicines and giving yourself your insulin shots. Connie is also learning it all with you. You both are definitely feeling the long road ahead of you, all the hard work that needs to continue, the learning of the meds, the breathing, the exercises, as well as the discipline and patience that is and will be needed by both of you.   The pot of gold at the end of the Rainbow is a better quality of life, one where you will be able to actually do things and not have to take that oxygen with you. You have a new set of lungs and now you have a new life ahead of you. Wednesday , April 18th is no different from any other day, filled with the walks, exercises, breathing, but today you seem a bit cranky. We were told you would be cranky (from your medicine), but then we expected you to be from time to time anyway. You have a big recovery time ahead of you, a lot of hard work and you get exhausted to the point of not wanting to do anything, even though you know you have to in order to make it to the next step. Thursday , April 19th PT walked with you to monitor your walking and breathing. They gave you a good report. Found out that you have too much fluid still around the new lungs so the tubes have to stay in another day. PT said your legs look good and the fluid in your feet was looking good. You walked all the way to the end of the hallway today. You were very exhausted after that. Friday , April 20th, the RN (Cathy

Bartos) came in and talked about home care, doctor appointments, and medicines. Gave us pamphlets to read. Today was a good day for you. You walked five times and did great with the spirometer. One of the doctors from Dr. Reddy's team stopped in to see you today and said considering what you went through during the surgery you have made great progress, and are looking really good. He told you, after you get the tube out you would be going home soon after.

Saturday, April 21st, more of the same. Walking, breathing, exercises. It's hard to believe it has been 19 days since your transplant. Today they said the tubes should come out soon. You are hoping things progress enough to be able to attend the support group meeting (coming up in about a week). It turned out I was released a day before the meeting, so ended up not going. I did go the following month. Deb, Rob and Dawn came up for a visit. We all went for a walk down the hallway with you, and Deb taped your progress. Today, Sunday, April 22nd they said they were going to do x-rays every other day now, also said you still had too much fluid around the lungs so the tubes were still not coming out. You had a little rattling going on in your chest so you were told to be sure to keep doing the breathing exercises. Monday, April 23rd you have one tube that still isn't ready to come out.

You walked the whole hallway without taking a break. That was very good. Your heart rate drops down low from time to time, and they need to give you magnesium when that happens. It's scary but they assured us that they expect to see this happen with transplant patients. That while it could be bad, they were on top of it. They assured us it would be okay. And it was. Still no tube out on Tuesday, April 24th, postponed another day. You are getting cranky about that because the area that the tube goes in is very sore. They keep telling you that when the tube comes out it will feel a lot better. So they keep getting your hopes up and it keeps getting delayed. But they needed to make sure you were ready. Wednesday, April 25th another day of the same, starting to get a very sore bottom from lying in the bed and sitting in the recliner for 24 days now. You were scheduled for a bronchoscopy today (one of five you would be having during the first year). Thursday, April 26th, was a big day—tubes came out. After taking the tubes out they took you down to x-ray. Everything is looking good and they say you might go home Friday or Monday. It looked like it was time for Connie to start organizing everything at the house she was staying at. Friday, April 27th you got the okay to go home. Connie got everything taken care of at the house, paid for the days she was there, cleaned up her room and packed everything up so she was ready to go when you were. By 7:00 p.m. you were on your way home. Kathy had been cleaning the house for the past week getting it ready for you to come home to. She washed all the bedding, curtains, dusted, and vacuumed. There were just a couple things that didn't get done, Deb, Rob, and Brandy went over and finished up with everything. Now you are home, but the hard work continues with PT two to three times a week, doctor appointments, a new routine of medicines and meals. You are on your own now, but phone numbers are at hand if the need arises.

The rest of this is my notes. Thank you Connie, and Debbie for keeping this record of events up to my discharge.

At this point, I will thank God, the doctors, and my family and friends for their prayers and support. There is one person I cannot, and never will, be able to thank enough, my Donor, my angel. She was a beautiful, young 15 year old girl. Her name was Heaven Leigh. She was autistic. She got very sick after ingesting a large amount of salt. Her sodium level went very high, and eventually went to her brain. She went into a coma, and never came out.

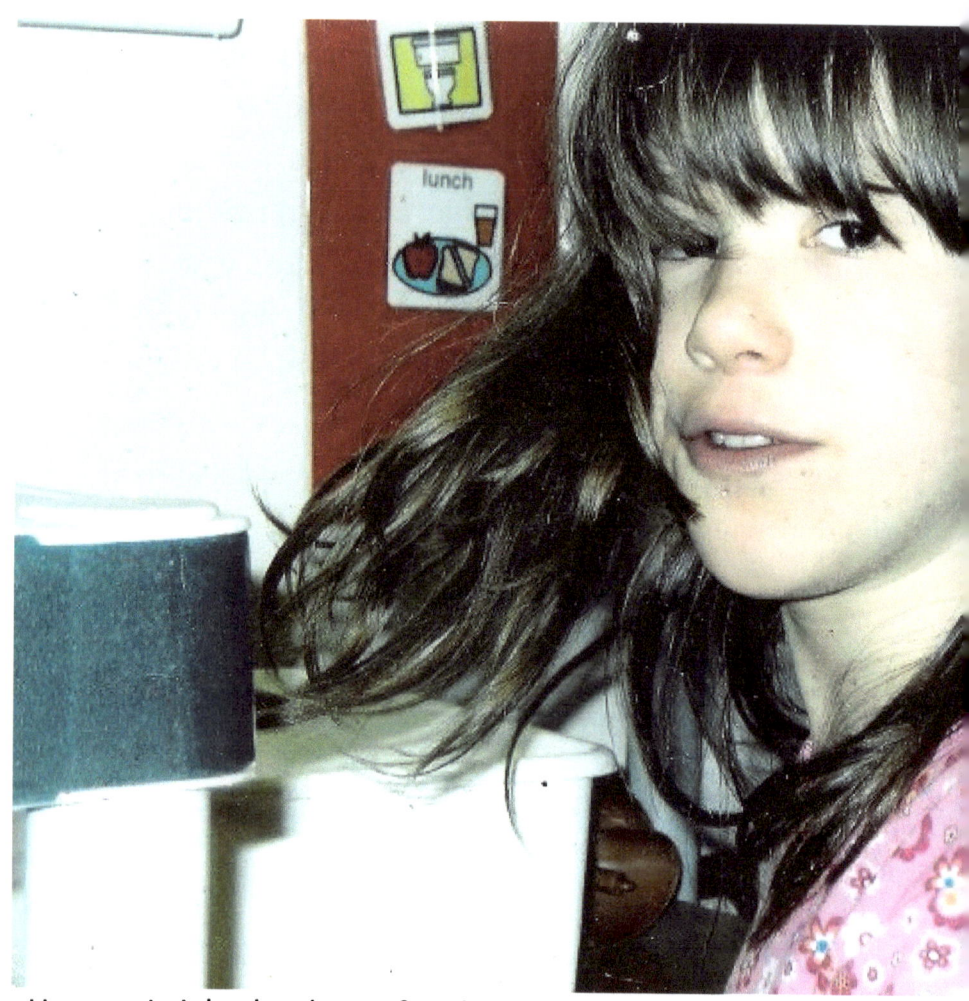

Heaven Leigh, thank you for the greatest gift a person could ever get, the Gift of Life. You are a part of me now, you are my Angel. I didn't know you, but I know you were loved, and will be missed, by many.

There have been a few issues since I've been home. Had stitches taken out of my ankle, where the tube for the echmo machine was inserted. A day or two later, the incision opened up. It had a lot of water draining from it, slowing the healing. This prevented me from starting pulmonary rehab until it heals. During a check up, Dr. Chan found I had a slight lung infection, so we stepped up one of my meds, the Bactrim. Still having a problem now and then with water retention, especially in my feet. Water retention, along with the steroids, has caused me to gain an unacceptable amount of weight. Wife and I are trying to change our eating habits, what we eat, and how much. Not easy, but I WILL get these extra pounds off. I'm also having a slight problem with my diabetes, every now and then my sugar levels go too high in the evening. Caused by my late night snacking, which I need to control, or stop.

Over all, I feel pretty good, a whole lot better than I did a few months ago. Physical therapist worked with me at home, teaching me upper and lower body exercises to help me build my strength and endurance back up. Home care nurse kept a very good eye on me, taking care of any questions or concerns that came up, and keeping records of all my vitals. She was also the go between with me and my lung Dr.

Late June, I think it was, I made contact with Heaven's mother. It was a brief letter exchange, arranged by The Gift of Life Foundation. We agreed we wanted to meet, and, also through Gift of Life, names, addresses, and phone numbers were exchanged. I called Heavens mother, Kimberly, and we agreed to meet the middle of

September, somewhere in St. Johns, about half way between us. I expect a lot of emotions flowing. When I received that first letter from Kim, there was a picture of Heaven Leigh enclosed. I looked at the picture and just lost it. I could not stop crying. I was told my donor was a man, a little younger than myself, a non smoker. I was very surprised when I seen it was a picture of a beautiful, young 15 year old girl. I called Gift of Life, to make sure they had sent me the right information. They assured me they had. I thank God for the gift Heaven has given me, and pray He blesses Heaven, and watches over her family.

  There is probably a lot more I could have added, so many more things happened during and after the surgery. I am waiting for the Dr. to set me up with a c-pap. Hopefully it will help me sleep at night. I have periods now and then when I have feelings of being out of breath, and I'm hoping the c-pap will help me with that. One of my bronchial tubes has closed about 40 percent, and may need a stent put in. That could be part of my breathing problem. It's going to be a long, slow recovery, and I know I have to work every day at getting back in shape, getting my health and strength back. I am in Pulmonary rehab, 3 times a week, and excersise the other days at home. I hope whoever reads this gets a little something out of my story. It was a major ordeal, I have no regrets about my decision to have the surgery. There were times i feared it would never happen, that I would never get "the call". It's over now, I'm back home, and the recovery begins. It has been 5 months since the surgery. About 2-3 weeks after I got home I started walking on the treadmill, real slow at first, and gradually increasing my speed and duration. I started pulmonary rehab , and will do that for about 4 months. The story isn't finished yet. I still have a lot of recovery ahead of me. I need to get back in shape, lose some weight, and build my strength back up. As long as I am on steroids, my weight will be a problem. I'm hoping better nutrition, and eating habits, will help me lose some pounds. I feel like most days are good days, but there are days once in awhile that are not so good. There are days when there are reactions to some of the meds, shaking, weight gain, water retention, irritability, so changes in meds are made. The Universith Of Michigan Medical Center has done an excellent job taking care of me. I can't say enough about them, including Doctors, nurses, techs, and anyone else that took care of me. Most of all I want to thank my wife Connie, who has been with me through all this, taking care of me, and encouraging me when I needed it most. Thanks to my sister Deb, who gave up a lot of her own time to stay with my wife, offering comfort and support. I also thank, with all my heart, all my family and friends, who offered prayers, support, best wishes, and also financial support. All these things were greatfully appreciated.

www.ingramcontent.com/pod-product-compliance
Lightning Source LLC
Chambersburg PA
CBHW042024200526
45159CB00035B/3043